The Anti-Inflammatory Diet Instant Pot Cookbook

Simple and Easy Instant Pot Recipes to Decrease Inflammation, Stay Healthy and Live Longer

Samanta Klein

Warning-Disclaimer

The purpose of this book is to educate and entertain. The author or publisher does not guarantee that anyone following the techniques, suggestions, tips, ideas, or strategies will become successful. The author and publisher shall have neither liability or responsibility to anyone with respect to any loss or damage caused, or alleged to be caused, directly or indirectly by the information contained in this book.

Contents

Introduction

Welcome to this Anti-Inflammatory Diet cookbook. So you have decided to start this diet and change your lifestyle. People, like you, opt this change for a number of reasons. Some do it for health reasons, some due to medical/dietary prescription, and some just want to lose weight and have better confidence in their bodies.

Yes – there are various sorts of rewards in choosing the anti-inflammatory diet and lifestyle. People who embark on this journey frequently get more than what they expect! Of course, no results are the same as we are all unique bodies and persons. HOWEVER, rest assured that you would definitely have a better well-being after adapting to an anti-inflammatory diet.

We are very glad that you have decided to make a lifestyle change with us. In this book, we will give you a perfect guide and ease your lifestyle and diet transition into a metamorphosis. In the next chapters, we will have a general discussion of the rules, strategies, and basic concepts related to a anti-inflammatory diet. After that, we will give you complete recipes so you do not have to worry about what to do next in your lifestyle change.

These recipes are selectively handpicked and tweaked with your well-being and comfort in mind. These are very easy to prepare in your Instant Pot pressure cooker and contain ingredients that may be already available in your cupboard. Most of all, they are delicious and perfect for all seasons.

Let's get started!

What is Inflammation and its causes?

Inflammation occurs when the body releases white blood cells to protect your body from unknown substances like foreign body contamination. It is specifically released to the injured or infected part of the body. Part of the body becomes red and swollen because the release of chemicals affects the blood flow.

There are good and bad aspects of inflammation. Yes, you read it right. Not all inflammation is bad. There are two types of inflammation and that is acute and chronic inflammation.

Acute inflammation occurs when you have sprain or sore throat. In this kind of inflammation, you are assured that the body is repairing itself and the inflammation will go away when your body is repaired. It seems that inflammation is good to the body, however there are times that the defense mechanism seems to crash. When it crashes, the inflammatory response is being set in motion even if there is no foreign body contamination. It is what happens when you have arthritis. Chronic inflammation is a different story. It takes several days and stays for a long time, leading to inflammatory diseases.

When the body has inflammation, it reacts to an injury, it send cells to fight the invading foreign objects. The immune system is being damaged and harmed. Instead of protecting the body, it causes harm and prtoblems in the body.

There are several factors that causes inflammation and one of the major cause of it is being linked to poor lifestyle choices.

- **Poor diet** – Are you fond of eating sugary foods? Is eating in fast-food chains one of your favorites? Eating unhealthy foods can trigger inflammation together with fat and increased blood sugar. A poor diet can result to higher weight or weight gain. It is known that having a higher body fat can result to several diseases that we don't want to have. It is important to eat healthy so we can decrease our body fat. When we improve our diet, we make it better by decreasing body's inflammatory response. This makes our body more efficient in managing potential complications of our weight gain.

- **Aging** – It is still controversial how aging affects inflammation, but according to science, the progressive degenerative process is tightly integrated with inflammation. As our body age, there are several body cells that is starting to die. They cannot regenerate itself. So when cells die, it becomes waste material or foreign substance in our body that can trigger inflammation.

- **Lack of physical activity** – Lack of physical activity can result to obesity and overweight. There is really a link between your lifestyle and your weight. Your unhealthy lifestyle can cause changes to your physiological response to inflammatory factors. Obesity, for instance, results in low-grade chronic inflammation.

- **Poor sleep** – Having a good night sleep is a good way to start our day but what if we are sleep deprived over a long period of time? Sleep deprivation can cause physical changes in our brain and our body that can lead to arthritis, periodontitis, and cancer. It can contribute to chronic diseases and mental health issues. Study shows that having less than 7-8 hours of sleep increases inflammation. It is also been linked in having chronic disease like heart problems, diabetes and hypertension.

- **Stress** – Emotional, physical or psychological stress is not good for you! All of that can raise cortisol in your body. Cortisol is a hormone that is produced by the adrenal glands. Higher level of cortisol can create inflammation. Studies found that chronic stress affects the body by altering immune cells activity. When you reduce stress, you live healthier.

- **Smoking** – We all know that smoking is not good for the body. Smoking affects and triggers immunologic response to vascular injury that is known to be linked with increased levels of inflammatory markers. Inflammatory markers are white blood cells and c-reactive protein.

There are a lot of factors affecting our body and its link to having inflammation. Thus it is necessary that we make to the things that we can control like turning to healthier options, changing our lifestyles and reducing our stress.

I believe that now that you have an idea on how chronic inflammation can harm your body, you are more interested to the recipes that can help you achieve a sustainable living.

Anti-inflammatory Diet

A diet that is focused on anti-inflammatory principles is very helpful and is highly recommended. There is a study that having this diet not only can protect you in diseases but also slow the process of aging by maintaining your blood sugar and increasing metabolism.

Optimize your health with anti-inflammatory diet. You should incorporate the anti-inflammatory principles:

1. **Fiber-rich foods** – Reduce inflammation by eating foods rich in fiber like fruits and vegetables. You can also get it from whole grains like oatmeal and barley.

2. **8 servings of fruits and vegetables everyday** – Increase your intake of garlic, onions, leek, broccoli, cabbage and cauliflower.

3. **Stay away from saturated fats** – Limit your red meat intake and use herbs and spices when you marinate meats to reduce the toxins formed when cooking.

4. **Avoid processed foods and refined sugar** – Artificial sweeteners and foods high in sodium are bad for your health and can trigger inflammation throughout the body. It can also cause other diseases like high blood pressure and increased insulin resistance.

5. **Avoid trans fats** – Saturated fats are no good but so are trans-fat. You need to avoid these kind of fats because the higher the trans-fat in the body, the higher the c-reactive protein that is a marker for inflammation in the body.

6. **Omega -3 fatty acids** – Consume foods that is rich in omegas-3 fatty acids like nuts, flax seeds, and beans. You can also take omega-3 supplement, but make sure that it is the best quality.

7. **Use oils with health fats** – Organic oils such as virgin and extra virgin olive oil are good choices. You can also use sunflower oil and canola. It has the best anti-inflammatory benefits.

Inflammation plays a part in so many diseases and has proven its association to immune system. We may not understand how it really works, but it is really visible by what you eat. Poor diet adds to its causes. Be empowered and limit the amount of inflammation in your body.

This cookbook is not only for people who already have inflammation or auto-immune disorders but also for people who wants to promote their overall well-being.

Now that you are familiar with inflammation and what it can do to our body, get know more about the Instant Pot. Instant Pot will be your partner in this endeavor to reduce inflammation.

The Instant Pot

The instant pot is a good substitute to your Pressure Cooker, Slow Cooker, Rice Cooker, Steamer, Sauté, Yogurt Maker and Warmer. It has smart programs that is user-friendly because of its easy-to-use control panel.

It is as easy as pressing a button. You can now prepare a variety of food for your family.

Features

- Has 10 safety mechanisms and UL safety certification.

- Energy efficient and kitchen friendly.

- Manual setting up to 120 minutes of cook time

- Multi-functional features from braising, pressure cooking, stewing, steaming, simmering, slow cooking, sauté/browning, fermenting, making yogurt and warming up foods.

- Has microprocessor inside that control time, cooking temperature and pressure. It has 14 cooking programs.

- Meal planner because you can use the feature delayed cooking up to 24 hours.

- Efficient and effective design because it can preserve the flavor and aroma of your food.

Instant Pot Functions

This cooker has different multi-functions specially designed for your needs. Below are the controls that you can use with this pot. It is very easy to use and so efficient. You will save dozen of time using this Instant Pot.

- **Keep Warm/Cancel** – This key is the standby state of the cooker. By pressing this key, you can cancel the program and activate the keep-warm program.

- **Soup** – This key is for soup and broth making. It is hassle free and saves time when using this control. Instant soup is on your table.

- **Meat/Stew** – This key is for meat and stew cooking. Enjoy a meal full of vegetables or meat cooked slowly in its broth.

- **Bean/Chili** – This key is for cooking beans and making chili. This is perfect for those who wants to take their beans in the next level.

- **Poultry** – This key is for cooking chicken, pork, goat, lamb, beef, etc. Savor the flavor of your favorite poultry meal.

- **Porridge** - This key is for making porridge using various grains such as oatmeal. Best enjoyed with milk!

- **Rice** – This key is for cooking white rice. No more mixing of rice. Just measure the right amount of cup of rice and water and wait for it to cook.

- **Multigrain** – This key is used for cooking other kind of rice like the brown rice and other grains like quinoa.

- **Steam** – This key is designed for steaming vegetables or your side dish.

- **Slow Cook** – This key is used if you want to turn your instant pot to a conventional slow cooker. The user can change the cooking time by pressing the "+" or "-".

- **Manual** – This key is being used to set time manually depending on what you need. You can set it until 240 minutes which is the maximum pressure cooking time.

- **Sauté** – This key is used for open lid sautéing, browning or simmering inside the inner pot.

- **Yogurt** – This key allows you to make yogurt, pasteurize mile and make fermented glutinous rice.

- **Timer** – This key is for delayed cooking. You can setup the time in the morning and schedule it in the afternoon so when you came home a meal will be ready for you.

Most of the controls can be adjusted depending on your need. You can slow it down or make it faster to achieve the style or the taste that you are looking for.

Benefits of using the Instant Pot

So, why should you buy the Instant Pot Pressure Coooker? Besides the fact that the Instant Pot has an incredible taste and flavor infusion technology that traps all of the cooking flavors and keeps the intensity of the taste, here are some other benefits that will definitely convince you why setting some money aside for this dream-come-true appliance of every homemaker is the best home investment to make this very instant:

It Saves Energy

Pressure cookers require less time to prepare food, which means that they use less energy to create equally delicious meals. Say goodbye to wasting your energy with your pots, pans, and burners, because once you start cooking with the Instant Pot you will drastically cut back on energy. That will not only keep more money in your pocket each month, but it will also keep your stove clean at all times – since you will rarely use it.

It is Super Time Efficient

The Instant Pot traps the heated steam that occurs inside the pot during the process of cooking and creates a high-pressure environment that contributes to quick cooking. But besides the fact that the steam and pressure will cook your meals 70 % faster than your stove, the efficiency of the Instant Pot is also in the preparation method. Because it requires no other pans, skillets, or woks, and uses a single-pot cooking method, the Instant Pot requires no special preparations, cooks without too much hassle, and will help you serve delicious meals in a snap.

It is Economical

Not only will the Instant Pot will save you time and money from energy, it will also allow you to cook inexpensive food to such a juicy and delightful perfection as if you used the most expensive cuts of meat and not those chops that were on sale.

It Preserves the Nutrients

Unlike the meals cooked with most of the traditional cookware, the Instant Pot leaves the nutrients intact. Due to the steam and pressure flow that is going on inside the Instant Pot during the cooking process, the food preserves its moisture and juiciness even after being cooked. The high-pressure environment locks inside all of the precious vitamins and nutrients, which adds healthier and more nutritious meals to your dinner table.

It Does Not Expose You to Harmful Substances

It is not uncommon for most cooking methods to deprive the foods of their wholesomeness and destroy the vitamins, minerals and other nutrients during the process of cooking, but they also create certain harmful compounds such as elements that can cause cancer or elevate the blood pressure. This is yet another reason why you should choose to cook your meals with the Instant Pot. Cooking under such pressure, the food is not only able to preserve its nutrients, but it is also not being exposed to harmful compounds.

It Has a Canning Option

Unlike the Instant Pot or other pressure cookers, this amazing extra-large kitchen appliance comes with the option for canning and preserving food. If you love using those extra fruits and veggies for creating some yummy canned good, then this is definitely the way to do it.

Cooking Tips for Your Instant Pot

The Instant Pot is not your regular kitchen appliance. It is in fact so versatile and multi-functional, and is basically a combination of many other appliances:

- It is a pressure cooker
- It is a slow cooker
- It is a sautéing pan and a stove top
- It is a rice cooker
- It is a steamer
- It is a warming pot
- It is a yogurt maker

If you have all of these appliances crowding your kitchen, replacing some of them with the Instant Pot is definitely the best choice.

However, it is its very versatility that intimidates people. If you are one of the many that simply cannot figure out how to get the most out of this device, then you might want to pay attention to these net revolutionary tips:

- You can cook frozen food without defrosting. All you have to do is simply add a couple of minutes to your cooking time.

- Do not force open the lid. You must allow for the pressure to be fully released before opening the lid. If the lid won't open, don't worry, it isn't stuck. That is just an indication that the Instant Pot pressure cooker is still pressurized and it still isn't safe to open the lid. Allow a few more minutes and try again.

– The Instant Pot is extremely safe to use, but only if you use it right. The best way to ensure that you will stay safe during releasing pressure and opening the lid is by ensuring that the venting knob is turned to the venting position, and by tilting the lid away from you when opening.

– The Instant Pot pressure cooker does not have a sautéing or browning function. With this appliance you can easily sauté food by choosing any of the given cooking options and cooking with the lid open. This makes the Instant Pot pressure cooker even more functional.

– Make sure not to overfill the Instant Pot. This will only increase the pressure and may even clog the valve. For best results, fill your Instant Pot up until it is 2/3 full. However, if you are cooking food that may raise or expand during the cooking process, fill it only halfway.

– Do not use too much liquid. Always follow the recipes until you have some experience under your belt and can create delicious recipes on your own. If you add more liquid than necessary, this will not only give your meals that 'rinsed' taste and dilute them, but it will also increase the time that is needed for the Instant Pot to go to pressure.

The Pressure Release

Luckily for every new user, the pressure valve of the Instant Pot has some pretty visible and easy-to-figure-out signs. IF you line up the circle symbol, you will lock the pressure in, and if you line up the symbol of the steam coming out, you are about to release the pressure.

Now, as to when you should use the quick release or natural pressure release method, here is what you should know.

Quick – The quick pressure release method means allowing the steam to come out quickly. There really isn't a rule, and you can basically use this method anytime, however, you do have to keep in mind that if the Instant Pot is filled with liquid and you release the steam out quickly, spillage will most likely occur.

This method is best to use after cooking meat, seafood, or veggies.

Natural – The natural pressure release method means just the opposite – allowing the steam to come out slowly. This method is best after cooking content that is starch-high, foamy food, or food with a large liquid volume.

Cooking Chart

It would be remiss not to mention this, I know, but since there is a pretty detailed information about the cooking time found in your Instant Pot manual, I will briefly explain the basis.

Here is how long you should cook food in your Instant Pot:

Fresh Fish– ready after 2-5 minutes of cooking

Vegetables – ready after 2-5 minutes of cooking

Chili – usual cooking time is 30 minutes

Beef Roast – usual cooking time is 35 – 40 minutes

Pork Roast – usual cooking time is 40 – 45 minutes

Whole Chicken – usual cooking time is 20 minutes

Juicy Ribs – usual cooking time is 20 minutes

If you are now excited to use your Instant Pot, it's time to explore the recipes provided for you. If you don't have an Instant Pot yet, get up now and buy one so you can get started in your kitchen!

Let's start cooking!

Cheesy Eggs and Arugula in Hollandaise Sauce

Preparation Time: 12 minutes / Servings: 4

Nutritional Info per Serving:

Calories 231, Carbohydrates 8.9 g, Fiber 0.1 g, Fat 14.6 g, Protein 15.4 g

Ingredients:

4 Whole-grain Bread Slices, chopped

4 Eggs, whisked

½ cup Arugula, chopped

4 slices of fresh Mozzarella Cheese

1 cup Water

1 ½ Ounces Hollandaise Sauce

Directions:

1. Place the steamer basket in your pressure cooker and pour the water inside.
2. Place the bread pieces in 4 ramekins.
3. Combine the eggs and arugula and divide this mixture between the ramekins.
4. Cover them with aluminum foil and close the lid of your pressure cooker.
5. Cook on MANUAL on high pressure for 5 minutes.
6. Then perform a quick pressure release by opening the valve to "venting".
7. Discard the foil and top with a slice of mozzarella and some hollandaise sauce.
8. Enjoy.

Cheese and Thyme Cremini Oats

Preparation Time: 30 minutes / Servings: 4

Nutritional Info per Serving:

Calories 266, Carbohydrates 31 g, Fiber 5 g, Fat 12 g, Protein 9 g

Ingredients:

8 ounces Cremini Mushrooms, sliced

14 ounces Chicken Broth

½ Onion, diced

2 tbsp olive oil

1 cup Steel-Cut Oats

½ cup grated Gouda or Cheddar Cheese

3 sprigs Thyme

½ cup Water

2 Garlic Cloves, minced

Salt and Pepper, to taste

Directions:

1. Add the butter in your pressure cooker, and press SAUTÉ.
2. Add onion and mushrooms and sauté for 3 minutes.
3. Add the garlic and sauté for one minute more.
4. Stir in the oats and cook for an additional minute.
5. Pour in the water, broth, and add thyme sprigs.
6. Season with some salt and pepper.
7. Seal the lid and cook on MANUAL on high for 12 minutes.
8. Once completed, let the pressure release naturally for 10 minutes, then perform a quick pressure release.
9. Serve immediately and enjoy.

Breakfast Vanilla Quinoa Bowl

Preparation Time: 13-15 minutes / Servings: 4

Nutritional Info per Serving per Serving:

Calories 186, Carbohydrates 35.7 g, Fiber 3 g, Fat 2.5 g, Protein 6 g

Ingredients:

1 cup Quinoa

2 tbsp Maple Syrup

1 tsp Vanilla Extract

1 ½ cups Water

A pinch of Sea Salt

Directions:

1. Place all the ingredients into your Instant Pot. Stir to combine well.
2. Seal the lid and cook on MANUAL on high for 1 minute.
3. Once ready, perform a quick pressure release by turning the valve to "venting".
4. Carefully open the lid, fluff with a fork and serve warm.

Giant Coconut Pancake

Preparation Time: 55 minutes / Servings: 4

Nutritional Info per Serving:

Calories 358, Carbohydrates 39 g, Fiber 18 g, Fat 15.3 g, Protein 16.1 g

Ingredients:

1 cup Coconut Flour

1 tsp Coconut Extract

2 tbsp Honey

2 Eggs

1 ½ cups Coconut Milk

1 cup ground Almonds

½ tsp Baking Soda

1 cup blackberries (optional)

Directions:

1. Whisk together the eggs and milk in a bowl. Gradually add the other ingredients, whisking constantly.
2. Grease a large ramekin or a heatproof container that will fit into the Instant Pot.
3. Pour the mixture into the greased ramekin. Pour 1 ½ cups of water into the Instant Pot and place the trivet inside.
4. Place the ramekin with the mixture on top of the trivet.
5. Seal the lid and turn the sealing vent to "sealing". Select MANUAL mode on high pressure and set the time to 45 minutes.
6. Once completed, perform a quick pressure release by turining the valve to "venting". Carefully open the lid. Loosen the edges then place the cooked pancake on a large plate. Serve with blackberries

Cherry and Chocolate Oatmeal

Preparation Time: 15 minutes / Servings:4

Nutritional Info per Serving:

Calories 283, Carbohydrates 54 g, Fiber 5.6 g, Fat 6 g, Protein 5 g

Ingredients:

3 ½ cups Water

⅛ cup Honey

1 cup oats (prefferably certified gluten-free)

3 tbsp Dark Chocolate Chips

1 cup Frozen Cherries, pitted

Directions:

1. Place all of the ingredients except the chocolate into your Instant Pot.
2. Stir well to combine. Seal the lid. Choose the MANUAL option and cook on high pressure for 12 minutes.
3. Once it goes off, perform a quick pressure release. Stir in the chocolate chips.

Sweet Potato, Tomato, and Onion Frittata

Preparation Time: 28 minutes / Servings: 4

Nutritional Info per Serving:

Calories 189, Carbohydrates 11.8 g, Fiber 2.6 g, Fat 11.3 g, Protein 10.9 g

Ingredients:

6 Large Eggs, beaten

1 Tomato, chopped

¼ cup Almond Milk

1 tbsp Tomato Paste

1 tbsp Olive Oil

2 tbsp Coconut Flour

1 ½ cups Water

5 tbsp chopped Onion

1 tsp minced Garlic Clove

4 ounces shredded Sweet Potatoes

Directions:

1. Whisk the wet ingredients together in a bowl (except the water).
2. Fold in the dry ingredients and stir to combine well.
3. Place the mixture in a baking dish that will fit into the Instant Pot.
4. Place a trivet in the pressure cooker and pour the water inside.
5. Place the baking dish in your pressure cooker on top of the trivet.
6. Seal the lid and turn the sealing vent to "sealing".
7. Cook for 18 minutes on MANUAL on high pressure.
8. Once completed, let the pressure release naturally for 10 minutes and serve hot.

Banana and Cinnamon French Toast

Preparation Time: 50 minutes / Servings: 6

Nutritional Info per Serving:

Calories 313, Carbohydrates 39 g, Fiber 2 g, Fat 15 g, Protein 8 g

Ingredients:

1 ½ tsp Cinnamon

¼ tsp Vanilla Extract

6 Whole-grain Bread Slices, cubed

4 Bananas, sliced

3 tbsp Brown Sugar

½ cup Almond Milk

¼ cup Pecans, chopped

3 Eggs

¼ cup Goat Cheese

2 tbsp cold and sliced Almond Butter

¾ cup Water

Directions:

1. Grease a 1 ½ quart baking dish and arrange half of the bread cubes.
2. Top the bread with half of the banana slices. Sprinkle half of the brown sugar.
3. Spread the goat cheese over the bananas. Arrange the rest of the bread cubes and banana slices over. Sprinkle with the remaining brown sugar and top with pecans. Top with the almond butter slices.
4. Whisk together the eggs, milk, cinnamon, and vanilla in a bowl. Pour the mixture over. Place the trivet into the Instant Pot and add the water.
5. Lower the baking dish inside the Instant Pot and close the lid. Cook on MANUAL on high pressure for 30 minutes. When ready, perform a quick pressure release.
6. Remove the lid carefully and quickly so the condensation doesn't drip on the French toast. Remove the baking dish using a sling or handles. Serve immediately.

Gluten-Free Tortellini Minestrone Soup

Preparation Time: 15 minutes / Servings:6

Nutritional Info per Serving:

Calories 245, Carbohydrates 34.2 g, Fiber 4.3 g, Fat 9.1 g, Protein 7.4 g

Ingredients:

1 Onion, diced

2 Carrots, diced

1 tbsp minced Garlic

2 tbsp Olive Oil

4 cups Veggie Broth

24 ounces jarred Spaghetti Sauce

1 tsp Brown Sugar

2 Celery Stalks, sliced

¼ tsp Black Pepper

1 ½ tsp Italian Seasoning

14 ounces canned diced Tomatoes

8 ounces Whole Wheat Tortellini

4 tablespoons grated Parmesan cheese, plus extra for garnish

Directions:

1. Add the olive oil to your Instant Pot and heat on SAUTÉ. Add the onions, garlic, celery, and carrots, and cook until they start to 'sweat'.
2. Stir in the rest of the ingredients. Seal the lid and set the Instant Pot on MANUAL on high pressure for 5 minutes.
3. Once cooking is complete, do a quick pressure release, then carefully open the lid. Check the tortellini. If they are too 'al dente' for your liking, you can continue boiling them with the lid off for a few more minutes.
4. Select Sauté and simmer on high until the desired texture is reached.Serve topped with Parmesan and basil.

Mushroom and Beef Stew

Preparation Time: 30 minutes / Servings: 4

Nutritional Info per Serving:

Calories 527, Carbohydrates 50 g, Fiber 6.3 g, Fat 17.7 g, Protein 44.6 g

Ingredients:

2 tbsp Canola Oil

1 tsp dried Parsley

1 Onion, chopped

1 ½ pound Beef, cut into pieces

4 Red Potatoes, cut into chunks

4 Carrots, cut into chunks

8 Button Mushrooms, sliced

10 ounces Golden Mushroom Soup

12 ounces Water

Directions:

1. Heat the oil in the pressure cooker on SAUTÉ.
2. Add the meat and brown it on all sides. Stir in the remaining ingredients.
3. Seal the lid and cook for 15 minutes on MANUAL mode on high pressure.
4. Allow for a natura pressure release for five minutes, then perform a quick release.
5. Carefully remove the lid and serve.

Lentil Soup

Preparation Time: 40 minutes / Servings: 4

Nutritional Info per Serving:

Calories 259, Carbohydrates 35.4 g, Fiber 16.3 g, Fat 7.5 g, Protein 13.3 g

Ingredients:

4 Garlic Cloves, minced

1 tsp Cumin

4 cups Veggie Broth

½ Onion, chopped

2 Celery Stalks, chopped

2 Carrots, chopped

1 cup dry Lentils

2 Bay Leaves

2 tbsp Olive Oil

Salt and Pepper, to taste

Directions:

1. Heat the olive oil in your pressure cooker on SAUTÉ.
2. Add onions, garlic, and carrots, and cook until they start to 'sweat'.
3. Add celery and sauté for one more minute.
4. Stir in the remaining ingredients.
5. Seal the lid and set the Instant Pot on MANUAL.
6. Cook on high pressure for 25 minutes.
7. When it is done, perform a quick pressure release.
8. Remove the lid and serve warm.

Irish Lamb Stew

Preparation Time: 40 minutes / Servings: 4

Nutritional Info per Serving:

Calories 321, Carbohydrates 28.8 g, Fiber 3.9 g, Fat 11.4 g, Protein 24.8 g

Ingredients:

1 pound Lamb, cut into pieces

1 Onion, sliced

2 tbsp Cornstarch or Arrowroot

1 ½ tbsp Olive Oil

2 Sweet Potatoes, cut into cubes

3 Carrots, chopped

2 ½ cups Veggie Broth

½ tsp dried Thyme

Directions:

1. Heat the olive oil in your pressure cooker on SAUTÉ.
2. Cook the lamb until browned on all sides.
3. Add all of the remaining ingredients, except the cornstarch, and stir well to combine.
4. Seal the lid and cook on MEAT/STEW mode for 10 minutes.
5. Let the pressure release naturally for 15 more minutes.
6. Whisk the cornstarch with a little bit of water and stir it into the stew.
7. Cook for another 3 minutes on MANUAL mode.
8. When it's done, perform a quick pressure release.
9. Serve and enjoy.

Pomodoro Soup

Preparation Time: 25 minutes / Servings: 8

Nutritional Info per Serving:

Calories 314, Carbohydrates 16 g, Fiber 2 g, Fat 23 g, Protein 11 g

Ingredients:

3 pounds Tomatoes, peeled and quartered

1 Carrot, diced

1 Onion, diced

¼ cup Fresh Basil

1 cup Coconut Milk

1 tbsp Tomato Paste

3 tbsp Butter

½ tsp Salt

½ tsp Pepper

29 ounces Chicken Broth

½ cup grated Parmesan Cheese

1 tsp minced Garlic

Directions:

1. Melt the butter in your Instant Pot and cook the onions, celery, and carrots until they start to 'sweat' on SAUTÉ.
2. Add garlic and cook for 30 more seconds.
3. Stir in the remaining ingredients, except the cream and cheese.
4. Close the lid and cook for 6 minutes on MEAT/STEW for 10 minutes.
5. Press STOP and wait for 5 minutes before doing a quick pressure release.
6. Stir in the coconut milk and parmesan cheese.
7. Serve and enjoy.

Pressure Cooked Chili

Preparation Time: 45 minutes / Servings: 4

Nutritional Info per Serving:

Calories 388.5, Carbohydrates 15.2 g, Fiber 2.9 g, Fat 27.6 g, Protein 22 g

Ingredients:

1 pound Ground Beef

½ cup Beef Broth

1 Onion, diced

1 tbsp Olive Oil

28 ounces canned Tomatoes

½ tbsp Cumin

1 ½ tbsp Chili Powder

1 tsp Garlic Powder

2 tbsp Tomato Paste

Directions:

1. Heat the olive oil in your Instant Pot on SAUTÉ mode.
2. Add the beef and cook the beef crumbling with a wooden spoon until it browns, about 4 minutes.
3. Add in the onion and cook for 2 more minutes.
4. Add cumin, chili, garlic powder, tomato paste, and cook for an additional minute.
5. Stir in the tomatoes and beef broth.
6. Seal the lid and cook for 25 minutes on MANUAL on high pressure.
7. Once if goes off, do a quick pressure release.
8. Serve and enjoy.

Pumpkin, Corn, and Chicken Chowder

Preparation Time: 15 minutes / Servings:4

Nutritional Info per Serving:

Calories 314, Carbohydrates 16.6 g, Fiber 5.8 g, Fat 21.1 g, Protein 14.7 g

Ingredients:

2 Chicken Breasts

2 cups Corn, canned or frozen

1 Onion, diced

¼ tsp Pepper

½ cup Coconut Milk

15 ounces Pumpkin Puree

29 ounces Chicken Broth

½ tsp dried Oregano

1 Garlic Clove, minced

Pinch of Nutmeg

Pinch of Red Pepper Flakes

2 Sweet Potatoes, cubed

2 tbsp Olive Oil

Directions:

1. Turn your Instant Pot on and press the SAUTÉ mode.
2. Add the olive oil and onion and sauté the onion until translucent.
3. Add garlic and stir-fry for 1 more minute.
4. Add pumpkin puree, the broth, and all the seasonings. Give it a good stir.
5. Stir in the potatoes and chicken, seal the lid and cook for 5 minutes on MANUAL on high pressure.
6. Once if goes off, do a quick pressure release and remove the lid.
7. Add the coconut milk and corn. Serve immediately.

Spicy Beef and Potato Soup

Preparation Time: 25 minutes / Servings: 8

Nutritional Info per Serving:

Calories 242.6, Carbohydrates 27.1 g, Fiber 4.2 g, Fat 9.3 g, Protein 14.7 g

Ingredients:

1 pound Ground Beef

1 tsp. olive oil

4 cups Water

24 ounces Tomato Sauce

2 cups Fresh Corn

2 tsp Salt

4 cups cubed Sweet Potatoes

1 Onion, chopped

½ tsp Hot Pepper Sauce

1 ½ tsp Black Pepper

Directions:

1. Select the SAUTÉ setting and add the olive oil and onion.
2. Sauté until the onion until tender, for about 2-3 minutes.
3. Add in the beef and cook until browned.
4. Then, stir in the remaining ingredients.
5. Seal the lid, select MANUAL and cook on high pressure for 10 minutes.
6. Once completed, allow for a natural pressure release, for 10 minutes.
7. Make sure to release any remaining steam before opening the lid.
8. Serve immediately.

Creamy Curried Cauliflower Soup

Preparation Time: 35 minutes / Servings: 4

Nutritional Info per Serving:

Calories 115.6, Carbohydrates 19.5 g, Fiber 4.1 g, Fat 2.8 g, Protein 2.8 g

Ingredients:

1 Cauliflower Head, chopped

1 tbsp Curry Powder

½ tsp Turmeric Powder

1 Sweet Potato, diced

1 Onion, diced

1 Carrot, diced

1 cup Coconut Milk

2 cups Veggie Broth

½ tbsp Coconut Oil

Directions:

1. Melt the coconut oil in your Instant Pot on SAUTÉ mode.
2. Add the onion and carrots and sauté for 3 minutes.
3. Add the rest of the ingredients.
4. Season with salt and pepper. Stir to combine well.
5. Close the lid, choose the MANUAL mode, and and cook at high pressure for 15 minutes.
6. Once cooking is complete, press Cancel and allo for a natural pressure release for 10 minutes.
7. Release any remaining steam before opening the lid.
8. Blend with a hand blender until smooth.
9. Transfer to a serving bowl and enjoy.

Hot & Spicy Shredded Chicken

Preparation Time: 1 hour / Servings: 4

Nutritional Info per Serving:

Calories 307.4, Carbohydrates 12.1 g, Fiber 1.2 g, Fat 10.2 g, Protein 38.3 g

Ingredients:

1 ½ pound boneless and skinless Chicken Breast

2 cups diced Tomatoes

½ tsp Oregano

2 Green Chilies, seeded and chopped

½ tsp Paprika

2 tbsp Coconut Sugar

½ cup Salsa

1 tsp Cumin

2 tbsp Olive Oil

Directions:

1. In a small bowl, combine the oil with all of the spices.
2. Rub the chicken breast with the spicy marinade.
3. Place the meat in your Instant Pot.
4. Add the diced tomatoes.
5. Close the lid and cook for 25 minutes POULTRY.
6. Transfer the chicken to a cutting board and shred it.
7. Return the shredded meat tot the Instant Pot.
8. Choose the SLOW COOK setting and cook for 30 more minutes.

Creamy Turkey and Mushrooms

Preparation Time: 40 minutes / Servings: 4

Nutritional Info per Serving:

Calories 192, Carbohydrates 5 g, Fiber 1 g, Fat 12 g, Protein 15 g

Ingredients:

20 ounces Turkey Breasts, boneless and skinless

6 ounces White Button Mushrooms, sliced

3 tbsp chopped Shallots

½ tsp dried Thyme

⅓ cup dry White Wine

⅔ cup Chicken Stock

1 Garlic Clove, minced

2 tbsp Olive Oil

3 tbsp Heavy Cream

1 ½ tbsp Cornstarch

Salt and Pepper, to taste

Directions:

1. Tie the turkey breast with a kitchen string horizontally, leaving approximately 2 inches apart.
2. Season the meat with salt and pepper.
3. Heat half of the olive oil in your Instant Pot on SAUTÉ mode.
4. Add the turkey and brown it for about 3 minutes on each side. Transfer to a plate.
5. Add the remaining oil, followed by the shallots, thyme, garlic, and mushrooms and cook for 5 minutes or until translucent.
6. Add white wine and scrape up the brown bits from the bottom.
7. When the alcohol evaporates, return the turkey to the pressure cooker and add the chicken broth.
8. Close the lid with the steam vent off and cook for 20 minutes on MANUAL.
9. Combine the heavy cream and cornstarch in a small bowl.
10. Carefully open the lid and stir in the mixture.
11. Bring the sauce to a boil, then turn the cooker off.
12. Slice the turkey in half and serve topped with the creamy mushroom sauce.

Teriyaki Chicken Under Pressure

Preparation Time: 25 minutes / Servings: 8

Nutritional Info per Serving:

Calories 352, Carbohydrates 31 g, Fiber 1.2 g, Fat 11.4 g, Protein 30.7 g

Ingredients:

1 cup Chicken Broth

¾ cup Brown Sugar

2 tbsp ground Ginger

1 tsp Pepper

3 pounds Boneless and Skinless Chicken Thighs

¼ cup Apple Cider Vinegar

¾ cup low-sodium Soy Sauce

20 ounces canned Pineapple, crushed

2 tbsp Garlic Powder

Directions:

1. Place the chicken in your Instant Pot.
2. Combine all of the remaining ingredients in a bowl.
3. Pour the sauce over the meat.
4. Seal the lid, select MANUAL and cook for 20 minutes on high pressure.
5. Once cooking is complete, select Cancel and perfome a quick release.
6. Serve and enjoy.

Fall-Off-Bone Drumsticks

Preparation Time: 45 minutes / Servings: 3

Nutritional Info per Serving:

Calories 454, Carbohydrates 6.7 g, Fiber 1.4 g, Fat 27.2 g, Protein 43.2 g

Ingredients:

1 tbsp Olive Oil

6 Skinless Chicken Drumsticks

4 Garlic Cloves, smashed

½ Red Bell Pepper, diced

½ Onion, diced

2 tbsp Tomato Paste

2 cups Water

Directions:

1. Heat the olive oil in your on SAUTÉ.
2. Add onion and bell pepper and sauté until softened, about 3 minutes.
3. Add garlic and cook until it becomes golden.
4. Season with salt and pepper, and mix gently.
5. Combine the tomato paste with water and pour it into the Instant Pot.
6. Arrange the drumsticks inside.
7. Seal the lid and cook for 15 minutes on POULTRY.
8. Once cooking is complete, release the pressure naturally for 10 minutes.
9. Taste for seasoning and serve.

Cherry Tomato, Olive, and Basil Chicken Casserole

Preparation Time: 30 minutes / Servings: 4

Nutritional Info per Serving:

Calories 337 Carbohydrates 11.8 g, Fiber 2.6 g, Fat 21.4 g, Protein 27 g

Ingredients:

8 small Chicken Thighs

½ cup Green Olives

1 pound Cherry Tomatoes

1 cup Water

A handful of Fresh Basil Leaves

1 ½ tsp minced Garlic

1 tsp dried Oregano

1 tbsp Olive Oil

Directions:

1. Heat the olive oil in your Instant Pot on SAUTÉ.
2. Cook the chicken about 2 minutes per side.
3. Place the tomatoes in a plastic bag and smash them with a meat pounder.
4. Remove the chicken from the cooker.
5. Combine tomatoes, garlic, water, and oregano in the pot.
6. Top with the browned chicken.
7. Close the lid and cook for 15 minutes on MANUAL mode on high pressure.
8. Let the pressure release naturally for at least 10 minutes, then release the rest of the pressure and takie the lid off. Stir in the basil and olives.
9. Stir and serve immediately.

Sweet and Smoked Slow Cooked Turkey

Preparation Time: 4 hours and 15 minutes / Servings: 4

Nutritional Info per Serving:

Calories 907.3, Carbohydrates 14.6 g, Fiber 0.6 g, Fat 50 g, Protein 95.2 g

Ingredients:

1 Turkey Breast (enough for 4 people, about 2 pounds)

2 tsp Smoked Paprika

1 tsp Liquid Smoke

1 tbsp Dijon Mustard

3 tbsp Honey

2 Garlic Cloves, minced

4 tbsp Olive Oil

1 cup Chicken Broth

Directions:

1. Brush the turkey breast with olive oil.
2. Set to SAUTÉ, and pour the oil.
3. Add in the turkey and brown it on all sides.
4. Place ½ cup chicken broth and all of the remaining ingredients in a bowl.
5. Stir to combine well.
6. Pour the mixture over the meat.
7. Seal the lid, set to SLOW COOK mode and cook for 5 to 6 hours.
8. After 2 hours, open the lid and pour the rest of the broth inside.
9. Let sit for at least 5 minutes before serving.
10. Serve and enjoy!

Chicken Piccata

Preparation Time: 20 minutes / Servings: 6

Nutritional Info per Serving:

Calories 318, Carbohydrates 15 g, Fiber 0.8 g, Fat 19.2 g, Protein 19.4 g

Ingredients:

6 Chicken Breast Halves

¼ cup Olive Oil

⅓ cup Freshly Squeezed Lemon Juice

1 tbsp Sherry Wine

½ cup Whole-Wheat Flour

4 Shallots, chopped

3 Garlic Cloves, crushed

¾ cup Chicken Broth

1 tsp dried Basil

¼ cup grated Parmesan Cheese

¼ cup Plain Yogurt

1 cup Pimento Olives minced

¼ tsp White Pepper

Directions:

11. Heat the olive oil in your Instant Pot on SAUTÉ mode.
12. Add the chicken and brown it on all sides. This will take 5 to 8 minutes.
13. Remove the chicken from the cooker. Add the shallots and garlic, and stir-fry them for couple of minutes. Add the sherry wine, broth, lemon juice, salt, olives, basil, and pepper. Return the chicken to the cooker.
14. Seal the lid and cook on MANUAL on High Pressure for 10 minutes.
15. Once ready, carefully open the lid. Stir in plain yougurt and parmesan.
16. Close the lid again and cook for an additional minute. Serve hot.

Sweet Gingery and Garlicky Chicken Thighs

Preparation Time: 45 minutes / Servings: 4

Nutritional Info per Serving:

Calories 786, Carbohydrates 80 g, Fiber 0 g, Fat 21 g, Protein 74 g

Ingredients:

2 pounds Chicken Thighs

½ cup Honey

3 tsp grated Ginger

1 tbsp plus 1 tsp minced Garlic

5 tbsp Brown Sugar

1 ¾ cup Chicken Broth

½ cup plus 2 tbsp Low-Sodium Soy Sauce

½ cup plus 2 tbsp Hoisin Sauce

4 tbsp Sriracha sauce

2 tbsp Sesame Oil

Directions:

1. Place the chicken on the bottom of your Instant Pot.
2. Combine the remaining ingredients in a bowl.
3. Pour the sauce over the chicken.
4. Seal the lid and cook for 40 minutes on MANUAL on high pressure.
5. Once if goes off, do a quick pressure release and open up.
6. Remove the chicken and transfer to a plate.
7. Serve and enjoy!

Creamy and Garlicky Italian Spinach Chicken

Preparation Time: 15 minutes / Servings:4

Nutritional Info per Serving:

Calories 455, Carbohydrates 3 g, Fiber 2 g, Fat 26 g, Protein 57 g

Ingredients:

1 cup chopped Spinach

2 pounds Chicken Breasts, boneless and skinless, cut in half

½ cup Chicken Broth

2 Garlic Cloves, minced

2 tbsp Olive Oil

¾ cup Heavy (Whipping) Cream

½ cup Sun-Dried Tomatoes

2 tsp Italian Seasoning

½ cup Parmesan Cheese

½ tsp Salt

Directions:

1. Rub the meat with the oil, garlic, salt, and seasonings.
2. Add the chicken in your Instant Pot, select SAUTÉ and brown it on all sides.
3. Pour the broth in, seal the lid and cook for 5 minutes on MANUAL on high pressure.
4. When it is done, release the pressure quickly, open the lid and add the cream.
5. Simmer for 5 minutes with the lid off, then add in the cheese.
6. Give it a good stir.
7. Stir in tomatoes and spinach and cook on SAUTÉ just until the spinach wilts.

Simple Cooked Whole Chicken

Preparation Time: 40 minutes / Servings: 4

Nutritional Info per Serving:

Calories 376, Carbohydrates 0 g, Fiber 0 g, Fat 30 g, Protein 25.1 g

Ingredients:

1 2-pound Whole Chicken

2 tbsp Olive Oil

1 ½ cups Water

Salt and Pepper, to taste

Directions:

1. Rinse the chicken and pat dry. Season with salt and pepper.
2. Press SAUTÉ and heat the oil in your Instant Pot and cook the chicken until browned on all sides.
3. Add the water in the pot then place the steam rack inside.
4. Place the chicken on the rack and seal the lid.
5. Select MANUAL and cook on high pressure for 25 minutes.
6. When it's done, do a quick pressure release.
7. Carefully take the chicken out of the pot and transfer to a serving plate.

Lamb Shanks Braised Under Pressure

Preparation Time: 50 minutes / Servings: 4

Nutritional Info per Serving:

Calories 804, Carbohydrates 19 g, Fiber 2.9 g, Fat 42.9 g, Protein 73.7 g

Ingredients:

4-6 Lamb Shanks

3 Carrots, sliced

2 Tomatoes, peeled and quartered

1 Garlic Clove, crushed

1 tbsp chopped Fresh Oregano

¼ cup plus 4 tsp Whole-Wheat Flour

8 tsp Olive Oil

1 Onion, chopped

¾ cup Red Wine

¼ cup Beef Broth

8 tsp Cold Water

Directions:

1. Place ¼ cup of the flour and the lamb shanks in a plastic bag.

2. Shake until you coat the shanks well. Discard the excess flour.

3. Heat 4 tsp of the oil in your Instant Pot on SAUTÉ mode.

4. Brown the shanks on both sides. Set aside.

5. Heat the remaining olive oil and sauté the onions, garlic and carrots for a couple of minutes.

6. Stir in tomatoes, wine, broth, and oregano.

7. Return the shanks to the cooker.

8. Seal the lid and cook for 25 minutes on MEAT/STEW mode.

9. Once ready, perform a quick pressure release.

10. Whisk together the remaining flour and water.

11. Stir this mixture into the lamb sauce and cook with the lid off until it thickens.

Saucy Beef Tips and Rice

Preparation Time: 40 - 45 minutes / Servings: 4

Nutritional Info per Serving:

Calories 358.5, Carbohydrates 64.1 g, Fiber 1.9 g, Fat 7.4 g, Protein 7.7 g

Ingredients:

2 tsp Salt

2 pounds Sirloin Steaks, cut into pieces

2 tbsp Vegetable Oil

2 Onions, chopped

½ tsp Paprika

¼ tsp Mustard Powder

½ tsp Black Pepper

3 tbsp Whole-Wheat Flour

2 Garlic Cloves, minced

4 cups cooked Brown Rice

10 ½ ounces Beef Consommé

Directions:

1. In a Ziploc bag, place the flour, mustard powder, salt, pepper, and paprika.
2. Add the beef cubes and shake the bag to coat them well.
3. Heat the oil in your Instant Pot on SAUTÉ and brown the meat on all sides.
4. Add the onions and garlic and sauté until translucent.
5. Stir in the beef consommé.
6. Close the lid and seal it. Select MANUAL mode and cook on high pressure for 20 minutes.
7. Release the pressure naturally for 10 minutes and simmer with the lid off until you reach your preferred consistency.
8. Serve over rice and enjoy.

Meatballs in Creamy Sauce

Preparation Time: 25 minutes / Servings: 4

Nutritional Info per Serving:

Calories 632.2, Carbohydrates 17 g, Fiber 1.9 g, Fat 43.9 g, Protein 41.1 g

Ingredients:

½ cup Coconut Milk

1 Onion, minced

1 ½ tbsp dried Thyme

1 pound Ground Beef

1 tbsp dried Oregano

8 ounces ground Pork

¼ cup Whole-Wheat Flour

½ tsp Salt

1 slice Whole-Wheat Bread

14 ounces Chicken Stock mixed with 14 ounces Water

1 Egg

¼ cup Olive Oil

½ cup Whipping Cream

¼ lb Cooked Egg Noodles

Directions:

1. Soak the bread in the milk in a bowl.
2. Add beef and pork and mix with your hands.
3. Stir in onion, thyme, oregano, egg, and salt. Form ¾-inch balls out of the mixture.
4. Heat the oil in your Instant Pot on SAUTÉ mode.
5. Whisk in the flour and gradually add the diluted chicken broth.
6. When the mixture begins to simmer, add the meatballs.
7. Seal the lid and cook on MANUAL mode for 10 minutes.
8. Perform a quick pressure release.
9. Carefully open the lid and stir in the cream and simmer with the lid off until the sauce thickens.
10. Serve over cooked noodles and enjoy.

Sloppy Joes and Coleslaw

Preparation Time: 30 - 35 minutes / Servings: 6

Nutritional Info per Serving:

Calories 180, Carbohydrates 18 g, Fiber 3.5 g, Fat g, Protein 3.5 g

Ingredients:

1 cup chopped Tomatoes

1 Onion, chopped

1 Carrot, chopped

1 pound Ground Beef

1 Bell Pepper, chopped

½ cup Rolled Oats

4 tbsp Apple Cider Vinegar

1 tbsp Olive Oil

4 tbsp Tomato Paste

1 cup Water

2 tsp Garlic Powder

1 tbsp Worcestershire Sauce

1 ½ tsp Salt

Coleslaw:

½ chopped Red Onion

1 tbsp Honey

½ head Cabbage, sliced

2 Carrots, grated

2 tbsp Apple Cider Vinegar

1 tbsp Dijon Mustard

Directions:

1. Heat the olive oil in your pressure cooker by setting SAUTÉ mode and brown the meat. Add the onions, carrots, pepper, garlic powder, salt, and sauté until soft.
2. Stir in tomatoes, vinegar, Worcestershire sauce, water, and tomato paste.
3. When the mixture starts to boil, stir in the oats. Seal the lid and cook for 15 minutes on MANUAL mode on high pressure.
4. Once the cooking is comple, perform a quick pressure release and let simmer with the lid off until thickened to your liking. Mix all of the slaw ingredients in a large bowl. Serve them with the slaw.

Worcestershire Pork Chops

Preparation Time: 35 minutes / Servings: 6

Nutritional Info per Serving:

Calories 785.2, Carbohydrates 25.9 g, Fiber 3.3 g, Fat 41.5 g, Protein 73.4 g

Ingredients:

1 Onion, diced

8 Pork Chops

¼ cup Olive Oil

3 tbsp Worcestershire Sauce

1 cup Water

4 Sweet Potatoes, diced

Directions:

1. Heat half of the oil in your pressure cooker on SAUTÉ.
2. Brown the pork chops on all sides and season with salt and pepper. Set aside.
3. Add the rest of the oil in the Instant Pot. Add onions and sauté for 2 or 3 minutes.
4. Add potatoes and stir in the water and Worcestershire sauce.
5. Return the pork chops to the cooker. Close the lid, press MEAT/STEW and cook for 15 minutes.
6. When cooking is complete, select Cancel and perform a natural pressure release.
7. This will take about 15 minutes.

Port Wine Garlicky Lamb

Preparation Time: 30 minutes / Servings: 4

Nutritional Info per Serving:

Calories 620, Carbohydrates 8.7 g, Fiber 0.5 g, Fat 34.9 g, Protein 60 g

Ingredients:

2 pounds Lamb Shanks

1 tbsp Olive Oil

½ cup Port Wine

1 tbsp Tomato Paste

10 Whole Garlic Cloves, peeled

½ cup Chicken Broth

1 tsp Balsamic Vinegar

½ tsp dried Rosemary

1 tbsp Olive Oil

Directions:

1. Heat the oil in the Instant Pot on SAUTÉ and brown the lamb shanks on all sides.
2. Add the garlic and cook until lightly browned, no more than 2 minutes.
3. Stir in the rest of the ingredients, except the oil and vinegar.
4. Seal the lid and cook for 20-25 minutes (depending on your preferred density) on MANUAL on high pressure.
5. When cooking is complete, release the pressure naturally for 10 minutes.
6. Remove the lamb shanks and let the sauce boil for 5 minutes with the lid off.
7. Stir in the vinegar and butter.
8. Serve the gravy poured over the shanks.

Veggie and Beef Brisket

Preparation Time: 1 hour and 30 minutes / Servings: 4

Nutritional Info per Serving:

Calories 400, Carbohydrates 10 g, Fiber 1 g, Fat 18 g, Protein 28 g

Ingredients:

4 Beef Tenderloin Filets

6 Sweet Potatoes, chopped

1 Onion, chopped

4 Bay Leaves

2 tbsp Olive Oil

2 cups chopped Carrots

3 tbsp chopped Garlic

3 tbsp Worcestershire Sauce

2 Celery Stalks, chopped

Pepper, to taste

1 tbsp Knorr Demi-Glace Sauce

Directions:

1. Heat 1 tbsp oil in your pressure cooker on SAUTÉ mode.
2. Sauté the onion until caramelized. Transfer to a bowl.
3. Season the meat with pepper, to taste.
4. Heat the remaining oil and cook the meat until browned on all sides.
5. Seal the lid and cook for one 1 minute on MANUAL mode on high pressure.
6. Release the pressure quickly and add the veggies and bay leaves.
7. Close the lid and cook for 15 more minutes. Transfer the meat and veggies to a serving platter. Whisk in the Knorr Demi-Glace sauce and simmer for 5 minutes until thickened.
8. Pour the gravy over the meat and enjoy.

Beef with Cabbage, Potatoes, and Carrots

Preparation Time: 1 hour and 5 minutes / Servings: 6

Nutritional Info per Serving:

Calories 712, Carbohydrates 55 g, Fiber 10.7 g, Fat 36.4 g, Protein 41.6 g

Ingredients:

6 Potatoes, peeled and quartered

4 Carrots, cut into pieces

2 ½ pounds Beef Brisket

1 Cabbage Head

3 Garlic Cloves, quartered

3 Turnips, chopped

2 Bay Leaves

4 cups of Water

Directions:

1. Pour the water into your Instant Pot.
2. Add the garlic and bay leaves.
3. Close the lid and cook for 45 minutes on MEAT/STEW.
4. Release the pressure quickly.
5. Add the veggies.
6. Close the lid and cook for 5 more minutes
7. Serve and enjoy.

Beef and Cheese Taco Pie

Preparation Time: 20 minutes / Servings: 4

Nutritional Info per Serving:

Calories 363, Carbohydrates 29 g, Fiber 6 g, Fat 19 g, Protein 25 g

Ingredients:

1 package Corn Tortillas

1 packet of Taco Seasoning

1 pound Ground Beef

12 ounces Mexican Cheese Blend

¼ cup Refried Beans

1 cup Water

Directions:

1. Pour the water in your Instant Pot.
2. Combine the meat with the seasoning.
3. Place one tortilla in the bottom of a pan and place it in your cooker.
4. Top with beans, beef, and cheese.
5. Top with another tortilla.
6. Repeat the process until you use up all of the ingredients.
7. The final layer should be a tortilla.
8. Seal the lid, and cook for 12 minutes on MANUAL on high pressure.
9. When it is done, let the steam release naturally for 5 minutes.
10. Then, release the remaining steam manually.
11. Remove the pan from the pot.
12. Serve hot.

Potted Rump Steak

Preparation Time: 30 minutes / Servings: 15

Nutritional Info per Serving:

Calories 615.8, Carbohydrates 11.1 g, Fiber 2.4 g, Fat 34.3 g, Protein 59 g

Ingredients:

3 tbsp Olive Oil

3 Bay Leaves

9 pounds Rump Steak

2 cups diced Celery

1 tsp Salt

3 Onions, chopped

2 cups sliced Mushrooms

18 ounces canned Tomato Paste

10 ½ ounces Beef Broth

1 ½ cups Dry Red Wine

Directions:

1. Heat the oil in your Instant Pot on SAUTÉ and brown the steak on all sides.
2. Add the vegetables and stir in all of the seasonings.
3. Combine the paste with the wine and broth.
4. Add this mixture to the cooker.
5. Seal the lid and cook for 35 minutes on MANUAL on high pressure.
6. Check the meat and cook for a little bit more if you don't like the density or you want your meat overcooked.
7. When the cooking is over, allow for a naturally release, for 10 minutes, then release the remaining steam manually.
8. Serve and enjoy.

Herbed Lamb Roast with Potatoes

Preparation Time: 30 minutes / Servings: 4

Nutritional Info per Serving:

Calories 739.2, Carbohydrates 1.3 g, Fiber 0.2 g, Fat 56.7 g, Protein 56.9 g

Ingredients:

6 pounds Leg of Lamb

1 tsp dried Sage

1 tsp dried Marjoram

1 Bay Leaf, crushed

1 tsp dried Thyme

3 Garlic Cloves, minced

3 pounds Sweet Potatoes, cut into pieces

2 tbsp Olive Oil

3 tbsp Arrowroot Powder

⅓ cup Water

2 cups Chicken Broth

Salt and Pepper, to taste

Directions:

1. Heat the oil in your Instant Pot on SAUTÉ mode.
2. Combine the herbs with some salt and pepper and rub the mixture into the meat.
3. Brown the lamb on all sides.
4. Pour the broth around the meat, close the lid, and cook for 60 minutes on MEAT/ STEW. Release the pressure quickly and add the potatoes.
5. Close the lid and cook for 10 more minutes. Transfer the meat and potatoes to a plate.
6. Combine the water and arrowroot and stir the mixture into the pot sauce.
7. Pour the gravy over the meat and potatoes and enjoy.

Clams in White Wine

Preparation Time: 17 minutes / Servings: 4

Nutritional Info per Serving:

Calories 224.4, Carbohydrates 5.8 g, Fiber 0.1 g, Fat 14.6 g, Protein 15.6 g

Ingredients:

¼ cup White Wine

2 cups Veggie Broth

¼ cup chopped Basil

¼ cup Olive Oil

2 ½ pounds Clams

2 tbsp Lemon Juice

2 Garlic Cloves, minced

Directions:

1. Heat the olive oil in your Instant Pot on SAUTÉ mode.
2. Add garlic and sauté for 2 minutes, .
3. Add wine, basil, lemon juice, and veggie broth.
4. Bring the mixture to a boil and boil for one minute.
5. Add your steaming basket, and place the clams inside.
6. Close the lid and cook for 5 minutes on MANUAL on high pressure.
7. Place the clams on a plate and drizzle with the cooking liquid.
8. Enjoy.

Lobster and Parmesan Pasta

Preparation Time: 25 minutes / Servings: 4

Nutritional Info per Serving:

Calories 441, Carbohydrates 44 g, Fiber 0 g, Fat 15 g, Protein 28 g

Ingredients:

6 cups Water

1 tbsp Whole-Wheat Flour

8 ounces dried Ziti

1 cup Plain Yougurt

1 tbsp chopped Tarragon

¾ cup Parmesan Cheese

3 Lobster Tails (about 6 ounces each)

½ cup White Wine

½ tsp Pepper

1 tbsp Worcestershire Sauce

Directions:

1. Add the water in the Instant Pot. Add the lobster tails and ziti.
2. Close the lid and cook for 10 minutes on MANUAL.
3. Do a quick pressure release.
4. Drain the pasta and set aside.
5. Remove the meat from the tails, chop it, and stir into the bowl with pasta.
6. Stir in the rest of the ingredients in the Instant Pot.
7. When the sauce thickens add the pasta and lobster.
8. Cook for another 1-2 minutes.
9. Serve and enjoy.

Shrimp and Egg Risotto

Preparation Time: 40 minutes / Servings: 6

Nutritional Info per Serving:

Calories 221, Carbohydrates 22 g, Fiber 1 g, Fat 10 g, Protein 13 g

Ingredients:

4 cups of Water

4 Garlic Cloves, minced

2 Eggs, beaten

½ tsp grated Ginger

3 tbsp Olive Oil

¼ tsp Cayenne Pepper

1 ½ cups frozen Peas

2 cups Brown Rice

¼ cup Soy Sauce

1 cup chopped Onion

12 ounces peeled and pre-cooked Shrimp, thawed

Directions:

1. Heat half of the olive oil in your Instant Pot on SAUTÉ mode.
2. Add the onions and garlic and cook for 2 minutes.
3. Stir in the remaining ingredients except the shrimp and eggs.
4. Close the lid and cook on RICE/RISOTTO for 20 minutes.
5. Wait about 10 minutes before doing a quick release.
6. Stir in the shrimp and eggs.
7. And let them heat for a couple of seconds with the lid off.
8. Serve and enjoy.

Almond-Crusted Tilapia

Preparation Time: 10 minutes / Servings: 4

Nutritional Info per Serving:

Calories 326.8, Carbohydrates 4.1 g, Fiber 2.8 g, Fat 14.9 g, Protein 46.1 g

Ingredients:

4 Tilapia Fillets

⅔ cup sliced Almonds

1 cup Water

2 tbsp Dijon Mustard

1 tsp Olive Oil

¼ tsp Black Pepper

Directions:

1. Pour the water in your Instant Pot.
2. Mix the olive oil, pepper, and mustard in a small bowl.
3. Brush the fish fillets with the mustardy mixture on all sides.
4. Coat the fish in almonds slices.
5. Place the rack in your pot and arrange the fish fillets on it.
6. Close the lid and cook for 5 minutes on MANUAL setting (may be more time of the fillets are thicker) on high pressure.
7. Do a quick pressure release and serve immediately.

Tuna and Pea Cheesy Noodles

Preparation Time: 17 minutes / Servings: 4

Nutritional Info per Serving:

Calories 430, Carbohydrates 42 g, Fiber 2 g, Fat 22 g, Protein 18 g

Ingredients:

1 can Tuna, drained

3 cups Water

4 ounces Parmesan Cheese, grated

16 ounces Egg Noodles

¼ cup Whole-Wheat Breadcrumbs

1 cup Frozen Peas

28 ounces canned Mushroom Soup

Directions:

1. Pour the water and noodles in your Instant Pot.
2. Stir in soup, tuna, and frozen peas.
3. Close the lid and cook for 5 minutes on MANUAL.
4. Release the pressure quickly. Stir in the cheese.
5. Transfer to a baking dish that can fit in your Instant Pot.
6. Sprinkle with breadcrumbs on top.
7. Place the baking dish in your Instant Pot.
8. Seal the lid and cook on MANUAL mode on high pressure for another 2 minutes.
9. Perform a quick pressure release.
10. Serve immediately.

Scallops & Mussels Cauliflower Paella

Preparation Time: 17 minutes / Servings: 4

Nutritional Info per Serving:

Calories 154.6, Carbohydrates 11.3 g, Fiber 3.7 g, Fat 4.5 g, Protein 7.1 g

Ingredients:

2 Bell Peppers, diced

1 tbsp Coconut Oil

1 cup of Scallops

2 cups Mussels

1 Onion, diced

2 cups ground Cauliflower

2 cups Fish Stock

A pinch of Saffron

Directions:

1. Press the Sauté button on the Instant Pot and melt the coconut oil.
2. Add the onion and bell peppers and cook for about 4 minutes .
3. Stir in scallops and saffron and cook for 2 minutes.
4. Stir in the remaining ingredients and close the lid.
5. Cook for 6 minutes on MANUAL mode on high pressure.
6. Once cooked, release the pressure manually for 10 minutes.

Lemon Sauce Salmon

Preparation Time: 10 minutes / Servings: 4

Nutritional Info per Serving:

Calories 493, Carbohydrates 6.3 g, Fiber 0.3 g, Fat 31.5 g, Protein 41.2 g

Ingredients:

4 Salmon Fillets

1 tbsp Honey

½ tsp Cumin

1 tbsp Hot Water

1 tbsp Olive Oil

1 tsp Smoked Paprika

1 tbsp chopped Fresh Parsley

¼ cup Lemon Juice

1 cup of Water

Directions:

1. Pour the water in the Instant pot then put the steamer rack in place.
2. Place the salmon on the steamer rack skin side down.
3. Seal the lid and cook for 3 minutes on MANUAL mode.
4. Meanwhile, in a bowl whisk together the remaining ingredients.
5. Once the cooking is over, release the pressure quickly, and drizzle the sauce over the salmon.
6. Seal the lid again and cook for 2 more minutes on MANUAL.
7. Then, perform a quick pressure release and serve immediately.
8. Serve and enjoy!

Vegetarian Spaghetti Bolognese

Preparation Time: 25 minutes / Servings: 8

Nutritional Info per Serving:

Calories 360, Carbohydrates 75 g, Fiber 8.2 g, Fat 2.3 g, Protein 15.1 g

Ingredients:

8 cups cooked Whole Wheat Spaghetti

1 cup Cauliflower Florets

 2 cups Shredded carrots

6 Garlic Cloves, minced

2 tbsp Tomato Paste

2 tbsp Agave Nectar

1 ½ tbsp dried Oregano

56 ounces canned crushed Tomatoes

2 tbsp Balsamic Vinegar

1 tbsp dried Basil

10 ounces Mushrooms

2 cups chopped Eggplant

1 cup Water

1 ½ tsp dried Rosemary

Salt and Black Pepper, to taste

Directions:

1. Add the cauliflower, mushrooms, eggplant, and carrots to a food processor and process until finely ground.
2. Add them to your Instant Pot. Stir in the rest of the ingredients.
3. Seal the lid and cook for 8 minutes on MANUAL on high pressure.
4. Once the cooking cycle has finished, release the pressure naturally for 10 minutes
5. Vent any remaining steam. Serve the sauce over the spaghetti.

Creamy Crabmeat

Preparation Time: 12 minutes / Servings: 4

Nutritional Info per Serving:

Calories 450, Carbohydrates 12.5 g, Fiber 0.3 g, Fat 10.4 g, Protein 40 g

Ingredients:

¼ cup Olive Oil

1 small Red Onion, chopped

1 pound Lump Crabmeat

½ Celery Stalk, chopped

½ cup Plain Yougurt

¼ cup Chicken Broth

Directions:

1. Season the crabmeat with some salt and pepper to taste.
2. Heat the oil in your Instant Pot on SAUTÉ mode. Add celery and cook for a minute. Add the onion and cook for 3 more minutes, or until soft.
3. Add the crabmeat and stir in the broth. Seal and lock the lid and set to STEAM mode for 5 minutes on high pressure.
4. Once the cooking is complete, do a quick release and carefully open the lid.
5. Stir in the yougurt and serve.

Cod in a Tomato Sauce

Preparation Time: 15 minutes / Servings:4

Nutritional Info per Serving:

Calories 251, Carbohydrates 3 g, Fiber 1 g, Fat 5.2 g, Protein 44.8 g

Ingredients:

4 Cod Fillets (about 7-ounce each)

2 cups chopped Tomatoes

1 cup of Water

1 tbsp Olive Oil

Salt and Pepper, to taste

¼ tsp Garlic Powder

Directions:

1. Place the tomatoes in a baking dish and crush them with a fork.
2. Season with some salt, pepper, and garlic powder.
3. Season the cod with salt and pepper and place it over the tomatoes.
4. Drizzle the olive oil over the fish and tomatoes.
5. Place the dish in your Instant Pot.
6. Close the lid and cook on MANUAL for 10 minutes.
7. Once the timer goes off, let the steam release naturally for about 10 minutes before releasing the remaining pressure manually.
8. Carefully open the lid and serve warm.

Mediterranean Salmon

Preparation Time: 15 minutes / Servings:4

Nutritional Info per Serving:

Calories 475.6 Carbohydrates 6.3 g, Fiber 2.7 g, Fat 31.5 g, Protein 42.9 g

Ingredients:

4 Salmon Fillets

2 tbsp Olive Oil

1 Rosemary Sprig

1 cup Cherry Tomatoes

15 ounces Asparagus

1 cup Water

Directions:

1. Pour the water in the Instant Pot and insert the steamer rack.
2. Place the salmon on the steamer rack skin side down, rub with rosemary, and arrange the asparagus on top.
3. Seal the lid and cook on MANUAL mode for 4 minutes.
4. Perform a quick pressure release and carefully open the lid.
5. Add in the cherry tomatoes on top and cook for another 2 minutes.
6. Perform a quick pressure release. Serve drizzled with olive oil.

Meatless Shepherd's Pie

Preparation Time: 17 minutes / Servings: 4

Nutritional Info per Serving:

Calories 224.4, Carbohydrates 5.8 g, Fiber 0.1 g, Fat 14.6 g, Protein 15.6 g

Ingredients:

⅓ cup diced Celery

1 cup diced Onion

2 cups steamed and mashed Cauliflower

1 tbsp Olive Oil

½ cup diced Turnip

1 ¾ cup Veggie Broth

1 cup diced Tomatoes

1 cup grated Potatoes

½ cup diced Carrot

½ cup Water

Directions:

1. Heat the olive oil in your Instant Pot on SAUTÉ mode.
2. Add the onion, carrot, and celery, and cook for 3 minutes.
3. Stir in turnips, potatoes, and veggie broth.
4. Seal the lid and cook for 10 minutes on MANUAL on high pressure.
5. Once it goes off, do a quick pressure release and open the lid
6. Stir in tomatoes. Transfer the mixture to 4 ramekins.
7. Top each ramekin with ½ cup of mashed cauliflower.
8. Place the trivet inside the Instant Pot and pour the water.
9. Seal the lid and cook for 5 minutes on MANUAL on high pressure.
10. When the timer goes off, allow for a natural pressure release for 10 minutes.
11. Then release the remaining pressure, carefully open the lid an serve.

Pressure Cooked Ratatouille

Preparation Time: 20 minutes / Servings: 4

Nutritional Info per Serving:

Calories 104, Carbohydrates 10.4 g, Fiber 0.5 g, Fat 7.2 g, Protein 1.5 g

Ingredients:

1 Zucchini, sliced

2 Tomatoes, sliced

1 tbsp Balsamic Vinegar

1 Eggplant, sliced

1 Onion, sliced

1 tbsp dried Thyme

2 tbsp Olive Oil

2 Garlic Cloves, minced

1 cup Water

Directions:

1. Add the garlic in a springform pan.
2. Arrange the veggies in a circle.
3. Sprinkle them with thyme and drizzle with olive oil.
4. Pour the water in your Instant Pot.
5. Place the pan inside.
6. Close the lid and cook for 10 minutes on MANUAL on high pressure.
7. Let the steam release naturally for about 10 minutes.
8. Carefully open the lid and serve immediately.

Bean and Rice Casserole

Preparation Time: 40 minutes / Servings: 4

Nutritional Info per Serving:

Calories 322, Carbohydrates 63 g, Fiber 9 g, Fat 2 g, Protein 6 g

Ingredients:

1 cup soaked Black Beans

5 cups Water

2 tsp Onion Powder

2 tsp Chili Powder, optional

2 cups Brown Rice

6 ounces Tomato Paste

1 tsp minced Garlic

1 tsp Salt

Directions:

1. Combine all of the ingredients in your Instant Pot.
2. Choose the MANUAL setting and seal the lid.
3. Cook for 35 minutes on high pressure.
4. Once the cooking is complete, let the pressure release for 5 minutes.
5. Then perform a quick pressure release.
6. Serve hot.

Potato Chili

Preparation Time: 30 minutes / Servings: 4

Nutritional Info per Serving:

Calories 297, Carbohydrates 53 g, Fiber 35 g, Fat 4 g, Protein 16 g

Ingredients:

15 ounces canned Black Beans, rinsed and drained

2 cups Veggie Broth

28 ounces canned diced Tomatoes

15 ounces canned Kidney Beans, rinsed and drained

1 Sweet Potato, chopped

1 Red Onion, chopped

1 Red Bell Pepper, chopped

1 Green Bell Pepper, chopped

1 tbsp Olive Oil

1 tbsp Chili Powder

¼ tsp Cinnamon

1 tsp Cumin

2 tsp Cocoa Powder

1 tsp Cayenne Pepper

Salt, to taste

Directions:

1. Heat the olive oil in your Instant Pot on SAUTÉ.
2. Add the onions, peppers, and potatoes. Cook until the onions become translucent.
3. Stir in the rest of the ingredients.
4. Seal the lid and cook on MANUAL mode for 12 minutes.
5. Once the cooking is complete, let the pressure release naturally for 5 minutes.
6. Serve hot.

Veggie Burger Patties

Preparation Time: 30 minutes / Servings: 4

Nutritional Info per Serving:

Calories 221, Carbohydrates 34.3 g, Fiber 6.5 g, Fat 7.1 g, Protein 3.4 g

Ingredients:

1 Zucchini, peeled and grated

3 cups Cauliflower Florets

1 Carrot, grated

⅔ cup Veggie Broth

2 cups Broccoli Florets

½ Onion, diced

½ tsp Turmeric Powder

2 tbsp Olive Oil

2 cups Sweet Potato cubes

¼ tsp Black Pepper

Directions:

1. Heat one tablespoon oil in your Instant Pot on SAUTÉ mode.
2. Sauté the onions for about 3 minutes.
3. Add the carrots and cook for an additional minute. Add potatoes and broth.
4. Close the lid and cook on MANUAL mode for 10 minutes.
5. Release the pressure quickly. Stir in the remaining veggies.
6. Close the lid and cook for 3 more minutes on POULTRY mode.
7. Mash the veggies with a masher and stir in the seasonings.
8. Let cool for a few minutes and make burger patties out of the mixture.
9. Heat the rest of the oil.
10. Cook the patties for about a minute on each side.

Fake Mushroom Risotto the Paleo Way

Preparation Time: 30 minutes / Servings: 4

Nutritional Info per Serving:

Calories 117.2, Carbohydrates 13.4 g, Fiber 5.5 g, Fat 11.1 g, Protein 2.8 g

Ingredients:

1 ½ head Cauliflower

2 cups sliced Mushrooms

1 Garlic Clove, minced

1 tsp dried Basil

1 Carrot, grated

1 cup Veggie Broth

1 tbsp Olive Oil

½ Onion, diced

Directions:

1. Cut the cauliflower into pieces and place them in your food processor.
2. Process until really ground (cauliflower rice). You should have about 6 cups of cauliflower rice.
3. Heat the oil in your Instant Pot set to SAUTÉ mode.
4. Sauté the carrots and onions for 3 minutes.
5. Add the garlic and cook for one more minute. Stir in all of the remaining ingredients.
6. Seal lid on pressure cooker and turn steam vent to Sealing.
7. Press MANUAL function and use the "+" and "-" buttons to adjust cook time to 5 minutes.
8. Immediately turn steam vent to Venting to Quick Release the pressure.
9. Carefully open the lid and serve immediately.

Spicy Moong Beans

Preparation Time: 40 minutes / Servings: 8

Nutritional Info per Serving:

Calories 328, Carbohydrates 62.4 g, Fiber 8.3 g, Fat 4.8 g, Protein 9.6 g

Ingredients:

1 tsp Paprika

2 tsp Curry Powder

4 cups Moong Beans, soaked and drained

1 Onion, diced

1 tsp Turmeric

Juice of 1 Lime

1 Jalapeno Pepper, chopped

1 Sprig Curry Leaves

4 Garlic Cloves, minced

2 tbsp Olive Oil

1 ½ tsp Cumin Seeds

2 Tomatoes, chopped

1-inch piece of Ginger, grated

Directions:

1. Heat the oil in the pressure cooker on SAUTÉ mode. Add the cumin seeds and sauté for about a minute and a half. Add the onion and cook until translucent, about 2 minutes.
2. Add garlic along with curry, turmeric, ginger, and some salt. Cook for one more minute. Stir in jalapeno, and tomatoes and cook for 5 minutes, or until soft.
3. Add the beans and pour water to cover the ingredients. Cover by at least 2 inches.
4. Add the lime juice and curry leaves and close the lid.
5. Select MANUAL mode and cook for 15 minutes on high pressure.
6. Once the cooking cycle has completed, allow pressure to release naturally.

Tamari Tofu with Sweet Potatoes and Broccoli

Preparation Time: 15 minutes / Servings:4

Nutritional Info per Serving:

Calories 250, Carbohydrates 22 g, Fiber 2 g, Fat 12 g, Protein 17 g

Ingredients:

1 pound Tofu, cubed

3 Garlic Cloves, minced

2 tbsp Tamari

2 tbsp Sesame Seeds

2 tsp toasted Sesame Oil

2 tbsp Tahini

1 tbsp Rice Vinegar

⅓ cup Vegetable Stock

2 cups Onion slices

2 cups Broccoli Florets

1 cup diced Sweet Potato

2 tbsp Sriracha

Directions:

1. Heat the sesame oil in your Instant Pot on SAUTÉ mode.
2. Add the onion and sweet potatoes and cook for 2 minutes.
3. Add garlic and half of the sesame seeds, and cook for a minute more.
4. Stir in tamari, broth, tofu, and vinegar.
5. Seal the lid and set steam vent to Sealing.
6. Select MANUAL mode and cook for 3 minutes on high pressure.
7. Release the pressure quickly, add thebroccoli and seal the lid again.
8. Cook for 2 more minutes.
9. Then, perform a qucik pressure release and open the lid.
10. Stir in sriracha and tahini before serving.

Tomato Zoodles

Preparation Time: 20 minutes / Servings: 4

Nutritional Info per Serving:

Calories 71.7, Carbohydrates 9.6 g, Fiber 2.5 g, Fat 3.8 g, Protein 1.9 g

Ingredients:

4 cups Zoodles

2 Garlic Cloves, minced

8 cups Boiling Water

1 tbsp Olive Oil

½ cup Tomato Paste

2 cups canned diced Tomatoes

2 tbsp chopped Basil

Directions:

1. Place the zoodles in a bowl filled with boiling water.
2. After one minute, drain them and set aside.
3. Heat the oil in your Instant Pot set to SAUTÉ.
4. Add garlic and sauté for about a minute, just until fragrant.
5. Add tomato paste and basil.
6. Stir in the zoodles, coating them well with the sauce.
7. Seal the lid and cook on MANUAL mode on High Pressure for one minute.
8. Turn steam vent from Venting to Quick Release the pressure.

Sweet Potato & Baby Carrot Medley

Preparation Time: 30 minutes / Servings: 4

Nutritional Info per Serving:

Calories 412.9, Carbohydrates 81.3 g, Fiber 13 g, Fat 7.5 g, Protein 7 g

Ingredients:

1 tsp dried Oregano

2 tbsp Olive Oil

½ cup Veggie Broth

1 Onion, finely chopped

2 pounds Sweet Potatoes, cubed

2 pounds Baby Carrots, halved

Directions:

1. Heat the olive oil in your pressure cooker on SAUTÉ.
2. Stir in the onions and cook for 2-3 minutes, until transclucent.
3. Add the carrots and cook for another 3 more minutes.
4. Add potatoes, carrots, broth and oregano.
5. Seal the lid and turn the steam vent to sealing.
6. Select MANUAL and cook for 10 minutes on high pressure.
7. Once the cooking is complete, allow pressure to release naturally, for 10 minutes.
8. Carefully open the lid and serve immediately.

Leafy Green Risotto

Preparation Time: 20 minutes / Servings: 6

Nutritional Info per Serving:

Calories 272, Carbohydrates 40 g, Fiber 3 g, Fat 11 g, Protein 6 g

Ingredients:

3 ½ cups Veggie Broth

1 cup Spinach Leaves, packed

1 cup Kale Leaves, packed

¼ cup grated Parmesan Cheese

¼ cup diced Onion

3 tbsp Olive Oil

2 tsp Olive Oil

1 ½ cups Arborio Brown Rice

4 Sun-dried Tomatoes, chopped

Pinch of Nutmeg

Salt and Pepper, to taste

Directions:

1. Heat the olive oil in your cooker on SAUTÉ.
2. Add the onions and cook until soft, about 2 minutes.
3. Add rice and cook for 3-4 more minutes.
4. Pour the broth over.
5. Close the lid and cook for 6 minutes on RICE/RISOTTO mode.
6. Do a quick pressure release and stir in the remaining ingredients.
7. Leave for a minute or two or until the greens become wilted.
8. Serve and enjoy.

Lemony and Garlicky Potato and Turnip Dip

Preparation Time: 15 minutes plus 2 hours in the fridge / Servings: 4

Nutritional Info per Serving:

Calories 143.5, Carbohydrates 12.3 g, Fiber 1.7 g, Fat 10.4 g, Protein 1.2 g

Ingredients:

3 tbsp Olive Oil

6 Whole Garlic Cloves, peeled

2 tbsp Lemon Juice

1 Turnip, cut lengthwise

1 Sweet Potato, cut lengthwise

1 cup Water

2 tbsp Coconut Milk

Directions:

1. Pour the water into your Instant Pot.
2. Place the potato, turnip, and garlic on the rack.
3. Close the lid and cook for 10 minutes on MANUAL mode.
4. Once the cooking has completed, turn off the Pot and let the pressure come down by itself.
5. Place the veggies in a food processor and add the remaining ingredients.
6. Process until smooth.
7. Transfer to a container with a lid.
8. Refrigerate for about 2 hours before serving.

Kale Chips with Garlic and Lime Juice

Preparation Time: 15 minutes / Servings:4

Nutritional Info per Serving:

Calories 66.5, Carbohydrates 7.7 g, Fiber 2.4 g, Fat 3.8 g, Protein 2.3 g

Ingredients:

1 pound Kale

½ cup Water

3 Garlic Cloves, minced

1 tbsp Olive Oil

2 tbsp Lime Juice

Directions:

1. Wash the kale and remove the stems.
2. Heat the oil in your Instant Pot on SAUTÉ mode.
3. Add garlic and cook for a minute, or just until fragrant.
4. Pack the kale well inside the cooker.
5. Close the lid and cook for 5 minutes MANUAL on High pressure.
6. Do a quick pressure release.
7. Transfer to a bowl. Drizzle the lime juice over.

Creamy Potato Slices with Chives

Preparation Time: 15 minutes / Servings:6

Nutritional Info per Serving:

Calories 168, Carbohydrates 31 g, Fiber 3 g, Fat 3 g, Protein 4 g

Ingredients:

6 Sweet Potatoes

⅓ cup Plain Yogurt

2 tbsp Cornstarch

1 tbsp chopped Chives

⅓ cup Almond Milk

1 cup Chicken Broth

Directions:

1. Peel and slice the sweet potatoes.
2. Coat them with salt, chives, and pepper.
3. Add broth and potatoes in your Instant Pot.
4. Seal the lid and set on MANUAL for 5 minutes.
5. Once the timer goes off, release the pressure quickly.
6. Carefully open the lid and transfer to a bowl.
7. Whisk the remaining ingredients into the cooking liquid in your pot.
8. Cook for one minute, stirring constantly.
9. Pour the sauce over the potatoes and enjoy.

Hummus Under Pressure

Preparation Time: minutes / Servings: 8

Nutritional Info per Serving:

Calories 161, Carbohydrates 20.2 g, Fiber 5.9 g, Fat 6.4 g, Protein 8 g

Ingredients:

1 Onion, quartered

1 Bay Leaf

2 tbsp Soy Sauce

¼ cup Tahini

¾ cup Garbanzo Beans

¼ cup dried Soybeans

¼ cup chopped Parsley

1 cup Veggie Broth

Juice of 1 Lemon

2 Garlic Cloves, minced

Directions:

1. Add garbanzo beans, soybeans, and broth in your Instant Pot.
2. Pour some water over to cover them by one inch.
3. Close the lid and cook for 15 – 20 minutes MANUAL mode.
4. Release the pressure naturally for 10 minutes.
5. Drain the beans and save the cooking liquid.
6. Place the beans along with the remaining ingredients into a food processor.
7. Process until smooth.
8. Add some of the cooking liquid to make the hummus thinner, if you want to.
9. Serve and enjoy!

Pressure Cooked Deviled Eggs

Preparation Time: 20 minutes / Servings: 4

Nutritional Info per Serving:

Calories 100, Carbohydrates 0.7 g, Fiber 0.2 g, Fat 7.9 g, Protein 6.4 g

Ingredients:

4 Eggs

1 tsp Paprika

1 tbsp light Mayonnaise

1 tsp Dijon Mustard

1 cup of Water

Directions:

1. Place the eggs and water in your Instant Pot.
2. Close the lid and cook for 5 minutes on MANUAL mode.
3. Let the pressure release naturally.
4. Place the eggs in an ice bath and let cool for 5 minutes.
5. Peel and cut them in half.
6. Whisk together the remaining ingredients.
7. Top the egg halves with the mixture and enjoy!

Mini Mac & Cheese

Preparation Time: 17 minutes / Servings: 4

Nutritional Info per Serving:

Calories 132, Carbohydrates 15.4 g, Fiber 1.6 g, Fat 5.4 g, Protein 7 g

Ingredients:

8 ounces whole-wheat Macaroni

¾ cup shredded Monterey Jack Cheese

2 cups Water

Directions:

1. Place the macaroni and water in your Instant Pot.
2. Press the RICE/RISOTTO setting and cook for 5 minutes.
3. Drain the macaroni and place them back in the pressure cooker,
4. Stir in the Monterey cheese and cook for 30 seconds until really well melted.
5. Divide between 4 small bowls.

Easy Street Sweet Corn

Preparation Time: 10 minutes / Servings: 6

Nutritional Info per Serving:

Calories 130, Carbohydrates 16 g, Fiber 2.4 g, Fat 5 g, Protein 9 g

Ingredients:

Juice of 2 Limes

1 cup grated Parmesan Cheese

6 Ears Sweet Corn

2 cups Water

6 tbsp Plain Yogurt

½ tsp Garlic Powder

1 tsp Chili Powder, optional

Directions:

1. Pour the water into your Instant Pot.
2. Place the corn in a steamer basket and inside the pot.
3. Close the lid and cook for 3 minutes on MANUAL mode.
4. Combine the remaining ingredients, except the cheese, in a bowl.
5. Release the pressure quickly and let cool for a couple of minutes.
6. Remove the husks from the corn and brush them with the mixture.
7. Top with parmesan and enjoy.

Full Coconut Cake

Preparation Time: 55 minutes / Servings: 4

Nutritional Info per Serving:

Calories 350, Carbohydrates 47 g, Fiber 7.5 g, Fat 14.1 g, Protein 7.5 g

Ingredients:

3 Eggs, yolks and whites separated

¾ cup Coconut Flour

½ tsp Coconut Extract

1 ½ cups warm Coconut Milk

½ cup Coconut Sugar

2 tbsp melted Coconut Oil

1 cup Water

Directions:

1. Beat the whites until soft form peaks.
2. Beat in the egg yolks along with the coconut sugar.
3. Stir in coconut extract and coconut oil.
4. Gently fold in the coconut flour.
5. Line a baking dish and pour the batter inside.
6. Cover with aluminum foil.
7. Pour the water inside your Instant Pot.
8. Place the dish in the pressure cooker.
9. Close the lid and cook for 45 minutes MANUAL mode.
10. Do a quick pressure release.
11. Serve and enjoy.

Peanut Butter Bars

Preparation Time: 55 minutes / Servings: 6

Nutritional Info per Serving:

Calories 561, Carbohydrates 61 g, Fiber 1.50 g, Fat 18 g, Protein 8 g

Ingredients:

1 cup Whole Wheat Flour

1 ½ cups Water

1 Egg

⅓ cup powdered Peanut Butter

⅓ cup Peanut Butter, softened

½ cup Almond Butter, softened

1 cup Oats

½ cup Packed Brown Sugar

½ tsp Baking Soda

½ tsp Salt

Directions:

1. Grease a springform pan and line it with parchment paper.
2. Beat together the eggs, powdered peanut butter, softened peanut butter, butter, salt, white sugar, and brown sugar.
3. Fold in the oats, flour, and baking soda. Press the batter into the pan.
4. Cover the pan with a paper towel and then with a piece of aluminum foil.
5. Pour the water into the pressure cooker and lower the trivet.
6. Place the pan inside and close the lid. Cook for 35 minutes on MANUAL mode.
7. Release the pressure naturally. Wait for about 15 minutes before inverting onto a plate and cutting into bars.

Oatmeal Chocolate Cookies

Preparation Time: 30 minutes / Servings: 2

Nutritional Info per Serving:

Calories 412, Carbohydrates 59 g, Fiber 1 g, Fat 20 g, Protein 6 g

Ingredients:

¼ cup Whole Wheat Flour

¼ cup Oats

1 tbsp Olive Oil

2 tbsp Packed Brown Sugar

½ tsp Vanilla Extract

1 tbsp Honey

2 tbsp Coconut Milk

2 tsp Coconut Oil

⅛ tsp Sea Salt

3 tbsp Bittersweet Chocolate Chips

Directions:

1. Combine all of the ingredients in a large bowl.
2. Line a baking pan with parchment paper.
3. Make lemon-sized cookies out of the mixture and flatten them onto the lined pan.
4. Add some water in your Instant Pot and lower the trivet.
5. Add the baking pan inside your pot.
6. Cook for 15 minutes on MANUAL mode on high pressure.
7. Release the pressure quickly, carefully open the lid and serve warm.

Easiest Pressure Cooked Raspberry Curd

Preparation Time: 25 minutes plus 1 hour in the fridge / Servings: 5

Nutritional Info per Serving:

Calories 249, Carbohydrates 48.4 g, Fiber 4.6 g, Fat 6.8 g, Protein 1.8 g

Ingredients:

12 ounces Raspberries

2 tbsp Almond Butter

Juice of ½ Lemon

1 cup Packed Brown Sugar

2 Egg Yolks

Directions:

1. Combine the raspberries, sugar, and lemon juice in your Instant Pot.
2. Close the lid and cook for a 1 on MANUAL mode.
3. Release the pressure naturally for 5 minutes.
4. Puree the raspberries and discard the seeds.
5. Whisk the yolks in a bowl.
6. Combine the yolks with the hot raspberry puree.
7. Pour the mixture in your pot.
8. Cook with the lid off for a minute on SAUTÉ mode.
9. Stir in the butter and cook for a couple more minutes, until thick.
10. Transfer to a container with a lid.
11. Refrigerate for at least an hour before serving.

Compote with Blueberries and Lemon Juice

Preparation Time: Active – 10 minutes, Passive – 2 hours and 40 minutes / Servings: 4

Nutritional Info per Serving:

Calories 220, Carbohydrates 61.2 g, Fiber 3.9 g, Fat 0.3 g, Protein 1.2 g

Ingredients:

2 cups Frozen Blueberries

2 tbsp Arrowroot or Cornstarch

¾ cups Coconut Sugar

Juice of ½ Lemon

2 tbsp Water

Directions:

1. Place blueberries, lemon juice, and sugar in your Instant Pot.
2. Close the lid and cook for 3 minutes on MANUAL mode.
3. Release the pressure naturally for 10 minutes.
4. Meanwhile, combine the arrowroot and water.
5. Stir the mixture into the cooked blueberries and cook until the mixture thickens.
6. Transfer the compote to a bowl and let cool completely.
7. Refrigerate for 2 hours.

Poached Pears with Orange, Cinnamon and Ginger

Preparation Time: 20 minutes / Servings: 4

Nutritional Info per Serving:

Calories 170.4, Carbohydrates 43.7 g, Fiber 5.2 g, Fat 0.6 g, Protein 1.1 g

Ingredients:

4 Pears cut in half

1 tsp powdered Ginger

1 tsp Nutmeg

1 cup Orange Juice

2 tsp Cinnamon

⅓ cup Coconut Sugar

Directions:

1. Combine the juice and spices in your Instant Pot.
2. Place the pears on the trivet.
3. Close the lid and cook for 7 minutes on MANUAL mode on high pressure.
4. Release the pressure naturally after 5 minutes.
5. Place the pears onto a serving plate.
6. Pour the juice over and serve.

Milk Dumplings in Sweet Cardamom Sauce

Preparation Time: 30 minutes / Servings: 20

Nutritional Info per Serving:

Calories 134, Carbohydrates 28.7 g, Fiber 0 g, Fat 1.5 g, Protein 2.4 g

Ingredients:

6 cups Water

2 ½ cups Packed Brown Sugar

3 tbsp Lime Juice

6 cups Almond Milk

1 tsp ground Cardamom

Directions:

1. Place the milk in a pot inside your Instant Pot and bring it to a boil.
2. Stir in the lime juice. The solids should start to separate.
3. Pour the milk through a cheesecloth-lined colander.
4. Drain as much liquid as you possibly can.
5. Place the paneer on a smooth surface.
6. Form a ball and then divide it into 20 equal pieces.
7. Pour the water in your pressure cooker and bring it to a boil.
8. Add the sugar and cardamom and cook until dissolved.
9. Shape the dumplings into balls, and place them in the syrup.
10. Close the lid and cook on MANUAL mode for about 4-5 minutes.
11. Let cool and then refrigerate until ready to serve.

Pressure Cooked Cherry Pie

Preparation Time: 45 minutes / Servings: 6

Nutritional Info per Serving:

Calories 393, Carbohydrates 70.6 g, Fiber 1.6 g, Fat 12 g, Protein 2 g

Ingredients:

1 9-inch double Pie Crust

2 cups Water

½ tsp Vanilla Extract

4 cups Cherries, pitted

¼ tsp Almond Extract

4 tbsp Quick Tapioca

1 cup Packed Brown Sugar

A pinch of Salt

Directions:

1. Add the water to the Instant Pot and place the steam rack on top.
2. Combine the cherries with tapioca, sugar, extracts, and salt.
3. Place one pie crust on the bottom of a lined springform pan.
4. Spread the filling over.
5. Top with the other crust.
6. Place the pan on the steam rack.
7. Seal the lid and cook for 18 minutes on MANUAL mode on high pressure.
8. Wait 10 minutes before releasing the pressure quickly.
9. Carefully remove the top so that any condensation doesn't drip on the pie, then carefully remove the pan using oven mitts or tongs.
10. Let it cool for at least 5 minutes before serving.

Crème Caramel Coconut Flan

Preparation Time: 30 minutes / Servings: 4

Nutritional Info per Serving:

Calories 107.8, Carbohydrates 16.5 g, Fiber 0 g, Fat 3.3 g, Protein 3.3 g

Ingredients:

2 Eggs

7 ounces Condensed Coconut Milk

½ cups Coconut Milk

1 ½ cups Water

½ tsp Vanilla

1 cup Packed Brown Sugar

Directions:

1. Place a pan with a heavy bottom in your Instant Pot.
2. Place the sugar in the pan. Cook until a caramel is formed.
3. Divide the caramel between 4 small ramekins.
4. Pour the water in the pressure cooker and lower the trivet.
5. Beat the rest of the ingredients together and divide them between the ramekins.
6. Cover them with aluminum foil and place in the pot.
7. Close the lid and cook for 5 minutes on MANUAL mode.
8. Release the pressure naturally for 10 minutes.

A Different Pumpkin Pie

Preparation Time: 30 minutes / / Servings: 4

Nutritional Info per Serving:

Calories 172.2, Carbohydrates 39.4 g, Fiber 3.6 g, Fat 1.9 g, Protein 2.8 g

Ingredients:

1 pound Butternut Squash, diced

1 Egg

⅓ cup Honey

½ cup Coconut Milk

½ tsp Cinnamon

½ tbsp Arrowroot or Cornstarch

1 cup Water

Pinch of Sea Salt

Directions:

1. Pour the water inside your Instant Pot. Place the butternut squash in the basket.
2. Seal the lid and cook for 4 minutes on MANUAL mode.
3. Whisk all of the remaining ingredients in a bowl.
4. Once the cooking is completed, perfrom a quick pressure release and drain the squash. Then, transfer to the milk mixture.
5. Pour the batter into a greased baking dish. Place inside the Insant Pot.
6. Seal the lid and cook for 10 minutes on MANUAL mode. Once it goes off, let the pressure release naturally for 5 minutes. Then perform a quick pressure release.
7. Very carefully remove the pan. Let it cool a few minutes before serving.

Your 7-Day Anti-Inflammation Meal Plan

Monday

Breakfast: Cheesy Eggs and Arugula in Hollandaise Sauce (p. 18)
Lunch: Gluten-Free Tortellini Minestrone Soup (p. 24)
Dinner: Sweet Potato & Baby Carrot Medley (p. 74)

Tuesday

Breakfast: Cheese and Thyme Cremini Oats (p. 19)
Lunch: Lentil Soup (p. 26)
Dinner: Curried potatoes with poached eggs

Wednesday

Breakfast: Breakfast Vanilla Quinoa Bowl (p. 20)
Lunch: Lemon Sauce Salmon (p. 60)
Dinner: Veggie Burger Patties (p. 69)

Thursday

Breakfast: Giant Coconut Pancake (p. 20)
Lunch: Saucy Beef Tips and Rice (p. 44)
Dinner: Tamari Tofu with Sweet Potatoes and Broccoli (p. 72)

Friday

Breakfast: Cherry and Chocolate Oatmeal (p. 21)
Lunch: Meatballs in Creamy Sauce (p. 47)
Dinner: Pressure Cooked Deviled Eggs (p. 80)

Saturday

Breakfast: Sweet Potato, Tomato, and Onion Frittata (p. 22)
Lunch: Pomodoro Soup (p. 28)
Dinner: Tuna and Pea Cheesy Noodles (p. 58)

Sunday

Breakfast: Banana and Cinnamon French Toast (p. 23)
Lunch: Fall-Off-Bone Drumsticks (p. 36)
Dinner: Pressure Cooked Deviled Eggs (p. 80)

Conversion Tables

Conversion Measurements in Cooking:

1 teaspoon		⅓ tablespoon	5 ml
1 tablespoon	½ fluid ounce	3 teaspoons	15 ml, 15 cc
2 tablespoons	1 fluid ounce ⅛ cup	6 teaspoons	30 ml, 30 cc
¼ cup	2 fluid ounces	4 tablespoons	59 ml
½ cup	4 fluid ounces	8 tablespoons	118 ml
1 cup	8 fluid ounces/ ½ pint	16 tablespoons	237 ml
2 cups	16 fluid ounces/ 1 pint	32 tablespoons	473 ml
4 cups	32 fluid ounces	1 quart	946 ml
1 gallon	128 fluid ounces		3785 ml, 3.78 liters
1 liter	1.057 quarts		1000 ml

Dry (Weight) Measurements (approximate):

1 ounce		30 grams (28.35 g)
2 ounces		55 grams
3 ounces		85 grams
4 ounces	¼ pound	125 grams
8 ounces	½ pound	240 grams
16 ounces	1 pound	454 grams
32 ounces	2 pounds	907 grams

| 1 kilogram | 2.2 pounds/ 35.2 ounces | 1000 gram |

Temperatures:

FAHRENHEIT (F)	CELSIUS (C)
250°F	120°C
300°F	150°C
325°F	165°C
350°F	180°C
375°F	190°C
400°F	200°C
425°F	220°C
450°F	230°C

Common Abbreviations for Measurements in Cooking:

COOKING ABBREVIATION(S)	UNIT OF MEASUREMENT
C, c	cup
g	gram
kg	kilogram
L, l	liter
lb	pound
mL, ml	milliliter
oz	ounce

t, tsp	teaspoon
T, TB, Tbl, Tbsp	tablespoon

Conclusion

Cooking with the Instant Pot takes some time to get used to, but there are many benefits such as reduced cooking time, healthier meals and saving money. And guess what, the Instant Pot is your best friend when trying to be on a specific cooking plan, because it's versatile and easy to clean. Today, there is so much you can do to improve on your health and follow an Anti-inflammatory diet experience.

I am sure you have enjoyed making these carefully selected anti-inflammatory recipes for comforting and healthy food. I hope these recipes have inspired you to get creative with your Instant Pot and that you are finally save from foods that cause you unnecessary inflamation and pain.

Made in the USA
Coppell, TX
23 November 2019